…… …… ..

Introduction: Unveiling the Measles Menace

In the annals of medical history, few adversaries
have wielded the same level of threat and
intrigue as the measles virus. Beyond its
innocuous-sounding name and characteristic red
spots lies a highly contagious and potentially
deadly pathogen that has plagued humanity for
centuries. From ancient civilizations to modern

societies, measles has left an indelible mark on the fabric of human health, challenging medical professionals, policymakers, and communities to confront its relentless onslaught.

In this introductory chapter, we embark on a journey into the heart of the measles menace, peeling back the layers of its enigmatic nature to reveal the stark realities of its impact on society. With a history dating back millennia, measles has long been recognized as a formidable adversary, capable of spreading with alarming speed and exacting a heavy toll on those it infects. From the crowded streets of urban centers to the remote corners of the globe, no population is immune to the threat posed by this insidious virus.

As we delve deeper into the complexities of measles, we confront not only its immediate health consequences but also its far-reaching implications for societal well-being. Past outbreaks in America and Africa serve as stark reminders of the havoc that measles can wreak when left unchecked, laying bare the vulnerabilities of even the most advanced healthcare systems. From the devastating loss of life to the economic upheaval wrought by prolonged outbreaks, the toll of measles extends far beyond the confines of the individual, reverberating through communities and nations alike.

Yet, amidst the shadows cast by this formidable foe, glimmers of hope emerge on the horizon. Advances in medical science and public health have paved the way for effective vaccines that hold the promise of stemming the tide of measles transmission. Through concerted efforts to expand access to immunization and bolster healthcare infrastructure, we stand poised to turn the tide against this ancient scourge, forging a path towards a future free from the specter of measles.

As we embark on this exploration of the measles menace, let us heed the lessons of the past, confront the challenges of the present, and chart a course towards a brighter, healthier future for all. Join us as we unravel the mysteries of measles and delve into the urgent imperative for collective action in safeguarding the health and well-being of generations to come.

… … …. …

Chapter 1: The History of Measles: From Ancient Times to Modern Eradication Efforts

Section 1: The Origins of Measles

The story of measles is as old as human civilization itself, with evidence suggesting that the virus has plagued populations since antiquity. In this section, we delve into the origins of measles, tracing its earliest known manifestations and the toll it exacted on ancient societies.

Measles is believed to have emerged thousands of years ago, likely originating from a closely related virus that infects animals such as cattle and dogs. As human populations expanded and began to settle in larger communities, measles found fertile ground for transmission, spreading rapidly among crowded populations with limited immunity.

The earliest recorded descriptions of a disease resembling measles date back to ancient civilizations such as the Egyptian, Greek, and Roman empires. Ancient texts and medical records contain references to outbreaks of a highly contagious illness characterized by fever, cough, and distinctive red spots on the skin—hallmarks of measles infection.

Throughout history, measles outbreaks have been documented in various regions of the world, often coinciding with periods of increased population density and travel. From the crowded cities of the Roman Empire to the bustling trade routes of the Silk Road, measles found ample opportunity to spread far and wide, leaving devastation in its wake.

Despite its ubiquity, the true nature of measles remained shrouded in mystery for centuries, with theories ranging from divine punishment to atmospheric influences proposed to explain its cause. It was not until the advent of modern microbiology in the 19th century that the viral nature of measles was definitively established, paving the way for groundbreaking advances in diagnosis, treatment, and prevention.

As we journey through the annals of history, we encounter tales of resilience and tragedy, as communities grappled with the relentless march of measles across the ages. From ancient pandemics that decimated populations to the dawn of vaccination and global eradication efforts, the story of measles is a testament to the enduring struggle between humanity and infectious disease.

… …. … … ..

Section 2: Past Measles Outbreaks in America

The history of measles in America is punctuated by a series of outbreaks and epidemics that have left indelible marks on the nation's public health landscape. In this section, we delve into the chronicles of past measles outbreaks in America, tracing their origins, impact, and enduring legacies.

The earliest recorded outbreaks of measles in America can be traced back to the colonial era, when European settlers brought the virus to the New World. The introduction of measles into indigenous communities had devastating consequences, as Native American populations lacked immunity to the newly introduced pathogen, leading to widespread illness and mortality.

Throughout the 19th and early 20th centuries, measles outbreaks continued to occur sporadically across the United States, fueled by factors such as urbanization, migration, and overcrowded living conditions. As cities grew and populations became more interconnected, measles found ample opportunity to spread, resulting in localized epidemics that swept through communities with alarming speed.

One of the most significant milestones in the history of measles in America occurred in the 20th century with the advent of measles vaccination. The introduction of the measles vaccine in the 1960s represented a monumental breakthrough in public health, offering a safe

and effective means of preventing measles
infection and its associated complications.

Despite the availability of the vaccine, measles
outbreaks continued to occur in the latter half of
the 20th century, fueled by factors such as
vaccine hesitancy, gaps in immunization
coverage, and international travel. In particular,
the 1989-1991 measles epidemic stands out as
one of the largest and most widespread
outbreaks in recent memory, resulting in tens of
thousands of cases and hundreds of deaths
across the United States.

In the decades since, concerted efforts have
been made to enhance measles vaccination rates
and strengthen public health infrastructure to
prevent future outbreaks. While progress has
been made in reducing the burden of measles in
America, recent challenges such as the
resurgence of vaccine misinformation and
pockets of under-vaccinated communities
underscore the ongoing importance of vigilance
and proactive measures to safeguard public
health against this persistent threat.

…… … … .

Chapter 2: Measles Epidemics in Africa:
Challenges and Lessons Learned

Section 1: Historical Context

The history of measles in Africa is a story of
both resilience and adversity, marked by
recurring epidemics that have posed significant
challenges to public health systems across the
continent. In this section, we delve into the
complexities of measles epidemics in Africa,
exploring their historical context, underlying
drivers, and enduring impacts.

Measles has long been endemic in Africa, with
periodic outbreaks occurring throughout history.
The virus thrives in communities where
vaccination coverage is low, poverty is
widespread, and healthcare infrastructure is
limited. As a result, Africa has borne a
disproportionate burden of measles-related
morbidity and mortality, particularly among
vulnerable populations such as infants, young
children, and malnourished individuals.

Section 2: Impact of Measles Epidemics

Measles epidemics in Africa have had far-reaching consequences, affecting not only individual health outcomes but also broader societal and economic dynamics. The toll of measles-related illness and death extends beyond the immediate clinical manifestations, encompassing long-term sequelae such as cognitive impairment, disability, and economic hardship.

Children are the primary victims of measles epidemics in Africa, accounting for the majority of cases and fatalities. The disease exacts a heavy toll on young lives, robbing them of their health, well-being, and future prospects. In addition to the direct impact on individuals, measles outbreaks can also strain healthcare systems, overwhelm medical facilities, and divert resources away from other essential health priorities.

Section 3: Challenges in Disease Control

Controlling measles epidemics in Africa poses unique challenges due to a confluence of factors, including inadequate healthcare infrastructure, limited access to vaccines, and socio-economic disparities. Weak health systems, fragmented immunization programs, and logistical barriers hinder efforts to achieve and sustain high vaccination coverage, leaving populations vulnerable to outbreaks.

Furthermore, misinformation, vaccine hesitancy, and cultural beliefs can undermine vaccination campaigns and fuel mistrust in public health interventions. Addressing these challenges requires a multi-faceted approach that combines targeted vaccination campaigns, community engagement, and health system strengthening initiatives.

Section 4: Lessons Learned and Future Directions

Despite the formidable challenges posed by measles epidemics in Africa, significant progress has been made in recent decades through concerted efforts to expand access to vaccination, strengthen surveillance systems, and improve outbreak response capabilities. However, the persistence of measles transmission in some regions underscores the need for sustained investment in immunization programs and health systems strengthening initiatives.

Looking ahead, achieving and sustaining measles elimination in Africa will require continued commitment from governments, international organizations, and civil society stakeholders. By learning from past experiences, adapting strategies to local contexts, and prioritizing equity and access, we can work towards a future where measles no longer poses a threat to the health and well-being of African communities.

. . . .

The Science Behind Measles

Section 1: Virology and Pathogenesis

Measles, caused by the measles virus (MeV), is a highly contagious viral infection that primarily affects the respiratory system. In this section, we explore the virology and pathogenesis of measles, shedding light on the intricate mechanisms by which the virus infects cells, evades the immune system, and spreads within the host.

The measles virus belongs to the Paramyxoviridae family and is characterized by a single-stranded RNA genome enclosed within a lipid envelope. Upon entry into the host's respiratory tract, MeV targets epithelial cells lining the airways, where it replicates rapidly and spreads to regional lymphoid tissues.

The hallmark clinical features of measles, including fever, cough, coryza, and conjunctivitis, arise from the systemic dissemination of the virus and the host's immune response to infection. MeV gains access to the bloodstream, leading to viremia and the characteristic maculopapular rash that typically appears several days after symptom onset.

Section 2: Immune Response to Measles

The immune response to measles is a dynamic interplay between the virus and the host's immune system, characterized by a complex series of interactions that influence disease outcomes. Here, we delve into the cellular and humoral components of the immune response to measles, highlighting key mechanisms of viral clearance, immunopathogenesis, and immune memory.

Upon encountering the measles virus, the host mounts an innate immune response characterized by the production of pro-inflammatory cytokines, activation of natural killer cells, and recruitment of dendritic cells and macrophages to the site of infection. These early immune responses play a crucial role in containing viral replication and initiating adaptive immunity.

The adaptive immune response to measles is orchestrated by T and B lymphocytes, which coordinate the elimination of infected cells and the production of virus-specific antibodies, respectively. Measles-specific T cells play a central role in clearing the virus from infected tissues, while neutralizing antibodies prevent viral spread and provide long-term immunity against re-infection.

Section 3: Complications of Measles

While measles is typically a self-limiting illness in immunocompetent individuals, it can lead to severe complications, particularly in young children, malnourished individuals, and those with underlying health conditions. Here, we examine the spectrum of measles complications, ranging from respiratory and neurological manifestations to immune-mediated sequelae.

Respiratory complications of measles include pneumonia, bronchitis, and croup, which can result from secondary bacterial infections or direct viral cytopathic effects. Neurological complications, such as encephalitis and subacute sclerosing panencephalitis (SSPE), are rare but can lead to long-term neurological sequelae or death.

In addition to acute complications, measles can also cause immune-mediated sequelae, such as measles-induced immunosuppression and measles-associated immune amnesia. These phenomena can increase susceptibility to secondary infections, compromise immune memory, and contribute to long-term morbidity and mortality.

Section 4: Vaccines and Immunization

Vaccination against measles has been instrumental in reducing the global burden of disease and preventing millions of deaths each year. In this section, we explore the history of measles vaccines, the principles of immunization, and the impact of vaccination on disease control and elimination efforts.

The first measles vaccine, developed by John Enders and colleagues in the 1960s, paved the way for the development of live attenuated vaccines that provide robust and durable immunity against measles. Mass vaccination campaigns, supported by organizations such as the World Health Organization (WHO) and the United Nations Children's Fund (UNICEF), have led to dramatic reductions in measles incidence and mortality worldwide.

Despite significant progress in measles control, challenges remain in achieving and sustaining high vaccination coverage, particularly in resource-limited settings. Vaccine hesitancy, logistical barriers, and outbreaks of vaccine-preventable diseases underscore the importance of strengthening immunization programs and addressing barriers to access.

By prioritizing equitable access to vaccines, strengthening healthcare infrastructure, and promoting vaccine acceptance and confidence, we can work towards a future where measles is no longer a threat to global health security.

… … …

Understanding the Measles Virus

Section 1: Introduction to Measles

Measles, also known as rubeola, is a highly contagious viral infection caused by the measles virus (MeV). In this section, we provide an overview of the measles virus, its classification, and its significance as a global health concern.

The measles virus belongs to the Paramyxoviridae family and is characterized by a single-stranded RNA genome enclosed within a lipid envelope. It is one of the most contagious pathogens known to humans, with a basic reproduction number (R0) ranging from 12 to 18, meaning that one infected person can potentially transmit the virus to 12 to 18 susceptible individuals.

Section 2: Transmission of Measles

Measles is primarily transmitted through respiratory droplets expelled when an infected person coughs, sneezes, or talks. In this section, we delve into the modes of transmission of the measles virus, including direct contact with infectious respiratory secretions and airborne spread in crowded settings.

The virus can remain viable in the air and on surfaces for several hours, making it highly infectious in enclosed environments such as schools, daycare centers, and healthcare facilities. Individuals who are not immune to measles, either through vaccination or previous infection, are at risk of contracting the virus when exposed to infected individuals or contaminated surfaces.

Section 3: Clinical Manifestations of Measles

The clinical manifestations of measles typically develop 10 to 14 days after exposure to the virus and progress through several stages. In this section, we explore the hallmark symptoms of measles, including fever, cough, coryza (runny nose), conjunctivitis (pink eye), and the characteristic maculopapular rash.

The prodromal phase of measles is characterized by the onset of non-specific symptoms such as fever, malaise, anorexia, and cough. As the illness progresses, Koplik spots—small white lesions on the buccal mucosa—may appear, followed by the characteristic maculopapular rash that spreads from the head and neck to the trunk and extremities.

Complications of measles, such as pneumonia, encephalitis, and otitis media, can occur, particularly in young children and immunocompromised individuals. Timely recognition of measles symptoms, prompt medical evaluation, and supportive care are essential for managing the illness and preventing complications.

… ….. ..

Complications and Long-Term Effects

Section 1: Measles Complications

Measles infection can lead to a range of complications, some of which can be severe or life-threatening. In this section, we discuss the potential complications associated with measles, including respiratory, neurological, and systemic manifestations.

1. Respiratory Complications: Measles can predispose individuals to respiratory complications such as pneumonia, bronchitis,

and laryngotracheobronchitis (croup). These complications can result from direct viral invasion of the respiratory tract or secondary bacterial infections.

2. Neurological Complications: Measles-associated encephalitis, characterized by inflammation of the brain, is a rare but serious complication of measles infection. Other neurological complications include seizures, acute disseminated encephalomyelitis (ADEM), and subacute sclerosing panencephalitis (SSPE), a rare and fatal progressive neurological disorder.

3. Systemic Complications: Measles can affect multiple organ systems, leading to systemic complications such as myocarditis (inflammation of the heart muscle), hepatitis (inflammation of the liver), and thrombocytopenia (low platelet count). These complications can contribute to the overall morbidity and mortality associated with measles infection.

Section 2: Long-Term Effects of Measles

While most individuals recover from measles without long-term sequelae, some may experience persistent health effects following acute infection. In this section, we explore the potential long-term effects of measles on various organ systems and overall health.

1. Immune Suppression: Measles infection can result in transient immune suppression, making individuals more susceptible to secondary infections in the weeks to months following acute illness. This phenomenon, known as measles-induced immune amnesia, can compromise the host's ability to mount an effective immune response to other pathogens.

2. Respiratory Effects: Individuals with a history of severe measles pneumonia may experience chronic respiratory symptoms, such as cough, wheezing, and exercise intolerance, due to lung damage and scarring. Long-term respiratory sequelae may impair lung function and quality of life in affected individuals.

3. Neurological Effects: Neurological complications of measles, such as SSPE, can have devastating long-term consequences,

including progressive cognitive decline, motor impairment, and ultimately, death. Survivors of measles-associated encephalitis may experience residual neurological deficits and cognitive impairment.

4. Psychosocial Effects: Measles infection and its complications can have psychosocial implications for affected individuals and their families, including psychological distress, social stigma, and financial burden. Long-term psychological support and rehabilitation may be necessary to address the emotional and social impact of measles-related disability.

… …. …. ..

Chapter 3: Measles and Society: Impact on Public Health

Section 1: Economic Burden of Measles Outbreaks

Measles outbreaks impose significant economic burdens on healthcare systems, governments, and affected communities. In this section, we examine the economic costs associated with measles outbreaks, including healthcare expenditures, productivity losses, and vaccination program costs.

1. Healthcare Expenditures: Measles outbreaks strain healthcare resources, leading to increased healthcare expenditures for diagnosis, treatment, and containment of the disease. Costs may include hospitalizations, outpatient visits, laboratory testing, and pharmaceutical interventions. The financial burden of measles-related healthcare services can escalate rapidly during large-scale outbreaks, overwhelming healthcare facilities and budgets.

2. Productivity Losses: Measles outbreaks can disrupt normal economic activities and productivity, as affected individuals may be unable to work or attend school due to illness or quarantine measures. Lost productivity stemming from absenteeism, reduced workforce participation, and caregiver responsibilities can have far-reaching economic consequences for individuals, families, and communities.

3. Vaccination Program Costs: Efforts to control measles outbreaks often require intensified vaccination campaigns, including mass vaccination initiatives, targeted outreach efforts, and supplemental immunization activities. These vaccination program costs encompass expenses related to vaccine procurement, distribution, administration, and monitoring. Additional resources may be needed to address vaccine hesitancy, improve vaccination coverage, and strengthen immunization infrastructure in high-risk populations.

4. Socioeconomic Disparities: Measles outbreaks disproportionately affect socioeconomically disadvantaged communities, exacerbating existing health inequities and socioeconomic disparities. Vulnerable populations with limited access to healthcare services, inadequate vaccination coverage, and suboptimal living conditions are at heightened risk of measles infection and its adverse consequences. Addressing socioeconomic determinants of health is essential to reducing the economic burden of measles outbreaks and promoting health equity.

By quantifying the economic costs of measles outbreaks, policymakers, public health officials, and stakeholders can better understand the financial implications of measles control and prevention efforts. Investing in comprehensive measles vaccination programs, outbreak response strategies, and health system strengthening initiatives is essential to mitigating the economic burden of measles outbreaks and safeguarding public health and well-being.

…. … … ..

Social and Cultural Factors Influencing Measles Transmission

Section 1: Community Dynamics and Measles Spread

1. Social Interactions: Measles transmission is facilitated by close social interactions, such as gatherings, communal living arrangements, and crowded settings where individuals have

prolonged contact with one another. High population density and social mixing patterns contribute to the rapid spread of the virus within communities.

2. Cultural Practices: Cultural beliefs, customs, and practices can influence measles transmission dynamics by shaping healthcare-seeking behaviors, vaccination attitudes, and disease management practices. Cultural factors may influence vaccine acceptance, healthcare utilization, and adherence to preventive measures, impacting measles control efforts.

3. Vaccine Hesitancy: Social and cultural factors play a significant role in vaccine hesitancy, contributing to suboptimal vaccination coverage and susceptibility to measles outbreaks. Misinformation, mistrust of healthcare authorities, religious or philosophical objections, and concerns about vaccine safety or efficacy can undermine vaccination efforts and fuel vaccine-preventable disease transmission.

4. Community Resilience and Engagement: Strong community engagement and resilience

are critical for effective measles control and prevention. Building trust, fostering partnerships with community leaders, and tailoring health promotion strategies to cultural norms and preferences can enhance vaccine acceptance and compliance with public health recommendations.

Section 2: Stigma and Discrimination

1. Stigmatization of Measles Cases: Individuals affected by measles may experience stigmatization and discrimination due to misconceptions about the disease, fear of contagion, and social stigma associated with vaccine-preventable illnesses. Stigmatizing attitudes and behaviors can exacerbate the psychosocial impact of measles on affected individuals and communities, hindering disease control efforts.

2. Marginalized Populations: Marginalized and vulnerable populations, including migrant communities, ethnic minorities, and underserved groups, may face heightened stigma and discrimination in the context of measles outbreaks. Social exclusion, blame, and

scapegoating can further marginalize already marginalized populations, impeding access to healthcare and support services.

3. Addressing Stigma and Discrimination: Combatting stigma and discrimination requires multifaceted approaches that promote empathy, education, and community solidarity. Public health messaging should emphasize empathy, compassion, and solidarity with individuals affected by measles, challenging stigmatizing narratives and fostering supportive social environments.

4. Promoting Equity and Inclusion: Measles control efforts should prioritize equity, inclusion, and social justice to address disparities in disease burden and access to healthcare. Culturally competent and inclusive approaches to health promotion, vaccination campaigns, and outbreak response are essential for reaching all segments of the population and reducing health inequities.

Understanding the social and cultural determinants of measles transmission is essential for designing contextually appropriate interventions, fostering community resilience, and promoting health equity. By addressing social and cultural factors influencing measles transmission, public health authorities can enhance the effectiveness of measles control strategies and protect vulnerable populations from vaccine-preventable disease.

… … ..

Measles' Toll on Healthcare Systems

Section 1: Healthcare Infrastructure Strain

1. Disease Burden: Measles outbreaks impose significant strain on healthcare systems, overwhelming medical facilities, and healthcare providers with a surge in patients presenting with measles-related complications. The increased demand for medical care, hospitalizations, and intensive care services can stretch healthcare resources to capacity, compromising the quality and accessibility of

healthcare services for both measles and non-measles patients.

2. Emergency Department Visits: Measles outbreaks often result in a sharp increase in emergency department visits, with individuals seeking evaluation and treatment for measles symptoms, complications, and vaccine-related inquiries. Emergency departments may experience overcrowding, extended wait times, and resource shortages during measles outbreaks, leading to delays in care and suboptimal patient outcomes.

3. Hospital Admissions: Severe cases of measles, including pneumonia, encephalitis, and other complications, may require hospitalization for supportive care, monitoring, and management of complications. Measles-related hospital admissions can strain inpatient facilities, intensive care units, and healthcare personnel, necessitating the allocation of additional resources to accommodate the influx of patients and maintain quality care standards.

4. Staffing Challenges: Measles outbreaks can pose staffing challenges for healthcare facilities,

as healthcare workers may be required to work
extended hours, provide specialized care for
measles patients, and respond to increased
demand for vaccination services and public
health interventions. Staff shortages, burnout,
and fatigue can compromise healthcare delivery
and exacerbate existing workforce challenges
within healthcare systems.

Section 2: Economic Costs and Financial
Impacts

1. Direct Healthcare Costs: Measles outbreaks
incur substantial direct healthcare costs,
including expenses related to medical
consultations, diagnostic tests, hospitalizations,
medications, and intensive care services. The
financial burden of measles-related healthcare
utilization can strain healthcare budgets,
insurance systems, and out-of-pocket
expenditures for affected individuals and
families.

2. Indirect Costs: Measles outbreaks also
impose indirect costs on healthcare systems,
economies, and society as a whole. Lost
productivity, absenteeism from work or school,

caregiver burden, and disruptions to routine healthcare services contribute to the economic impact of measles outbreaks, affecting individuals, employers, businesses, and governments.

3. Healthcare System Resilience: Measles outbreaks test the resilience of healthcare systems, highlighting vulnerabilities in healthcare infrastructure, emergency response capabilities, and pandemic preparedness. Strengthening healthcare system resilience through investments in infrastructure, workforce development, surveillance, and outbreak response capacity is essential for mitigating the impact of measles outbreaks and other public health emergencies.

4. Long-Term Consequences: The long-term consequences of measles outbreaks extend beyond the immediate healthcare crisis, with lasting effects on population health, healthcare delivery, and economic stability. Addressing the root causes of measles transmission, improving vaccination coverage, and investing in healthcare system strengthening are essential

for building resilience to future outbreaks and safeguarding public health.

. . . .

Chapter 4: Combatting Measles: Prevention and Control Measures

Section 1: Vaccination Campaigns

1. Importance of Vaccination: Vaccination remains the most effective strategy for preventing measles transmission, reducing morbidity and mortality, and achieving measles elimination goals. Vaccination campaigns aim to immunize individuals against measles virus, thereby conferring immunity and contributing to herd immunity within communities.

2. Routine Immunization Programs: National immunization programs prioritize routine measles vaccination as part of childhood immunization schedules, providing timely doses

of measles-containing vaccines (MCV) to infants and children to ensure protection against measles infection. Routine immunization coverage, vaccine availability, and vaccine uptake are critical components of measles prevention efforts.

3. Catch-Up Vaccination: Catch-up vaccination campaigns target susceptible populations, including unvaccinated individuals, under-vaccinated groups, and older age cohorts who may have missed routine vaccination opportunities. Catch-up campaigns seek to close immunity gaps, increase population immunity, and prevent measles outbreaks by reaching individuals who are at risk of measles infection.

4. Mass Vaccination Campaigns: In response to measles outbreaks or heightened transmission risk, mass vaccination campaigns may be implemented to rapidly immunize large segments of the population, particularly in high-risk settings or communities with low vaccination coverage. Mass vaccination campaigns involve coordinated efforts to deliver measles vaccines to targeted populations, including schools, healthcare

facilities, community centers, and mobile vaccination clinics.

Section 2: Herd Immunity

1. Concept of Herd Immunity: Herd immunity, also known as community immunity, refers to the indirect protection conferred on individuals within a population when a sufficiently high proportion of the population is immune to a contagious disease, such as measles. Herd immunity reduces the likelihood of disease transmission and provides protection to vulnerable individuals who may be unable to receive vaccination.

2. Threshold for Herd Immunity: The threshold for achieving herd immunity against measles varies depending on the basic reproduction number ($R0$) of the virus, which represents the average number of secondary cases generated by a single infected individual in a susceptible population. For measles, which has a high $R0$ value, herd immunity typically requires vaccination coverage of 90% to 95% or higher to interrupt transmission chains and prevent sustained outbreaks.

3. Role of Vaccination Coverage: Maintaining high vaccination coverage levels is essential for sustaining herd immunity and preventing measles resurgence. Declines in vaccination coverage, vaccine hesitancy, and gaps in immunization programs can undermine herd immunity, increase susceptibility to measles outbreaks, and compromise population-level protection against measles infection.

4. Challenges and Strategies: Achieving and maintaining herd immunity against measles requires coordinated efforts to address barriers to vaccination, enhance vaccine access and affordability, counter misinformation and vaccine hesitancy, and strengthen immunization systems. Multisectoral collaboration, community engagement, and evidence-based interventions are key strategies for promoting vaccine acceptance and achieving sustainable measles control.

… … …. ….

Strategies for Measles Surveillance and Response

Section 1: Measles Surveillance

1. Importance of Surveillance: Effective surveillance systems play a crucial role in monitoring measles incidence, detecting outbreaks, and guiding public health interventions. Measles surveillance involves the systematic collection, analysis, and interpretation of data on suspected and confirmed cases of measles to inform disease control efforts.

2. Case Definition and Reporting: Standardized case definitions for suspected, probable, and confirmed measles cases facilitate consistent reporting and surveillance across regions. Healthcare providers, laboratories, and public health authorities report suspected cases to designated surveillance systems, triggering investigation and response activities.

3. Laboratory Confirmation: Laboratory testing, including serological assays and molecular diagnostics, is essential for confirming measles cases, differentiating measles from other febrile rash illnesses, and identifying measles virus genotypes. Timely and accurate laboratory diagnosis enhances surveillance accuracy and enables targeted public health interventions.

4. Sentinel Surveillance: Sentinel surveillance systems involve the systematic collection of data from selected healthcare facilities, clinics, or laboratories to monitor measles trends, detect outbreaks, and assess vaccination coverage. Sentinel sites provide representative data on measles incidence and help evaluate the effectiveness of vaccination programs.

Section 2: Outbreak Response

1. Rapid Response Teams: Rapid response teams comprising epidemiologists, healthcare workers, and public health officials are mobilized to investigate suspected measles outbreaks, implement control measures, and mitigate transmission risks. Rapid response teams conduct case investigations, contact

tracing, and vaccination campaigns to contain outbreaks and prevent further spread.

2. Vaccination Strategies: Vaccination is a cornerstone of measles outbreak response, aiming to rapidly increase population immunity and interrupt transmission chains. Outbreak response vaccination campaigns target affected communities, high-risk settings, and susceptible populations to ensure timely administration of measles-containing vaccines (MCV) and boost immunity levels.

3. Case Management and Isolation: Prompt identification, diagnosis, and isolation of measles cases are critical for preventing secondary transmission and controlling outbreaks. Infected individuals are advised to self-isolate to minimize exposure to susceptible contacts, while healthcare facilities implement infection control measures to prevent nosocomial spread.

4. Public Health Communication: Clear and timely communication with affected communities, healthcare providers, and the public is essential for promoting awareness,

enhancing surveillance, and fostering community participation in outbreak response efforts. Public health authorities utilize various communication channels to disseminate information, address concerns, and promote vaccination uptake during measles outbreaks.

....

Addressing Vaccine Hesitancy and Misinformation

Section 1: Understanding Vaccine Hesitancy

1. Factors Contributing to Vaccine Hesitancy: Vaccine hesitancy encompasses a spectrum of attitudes and beliefs towards vaccination, influenced by diverse individual, societal, and contextual factors. Understanding the drivers of vaccine hesitancy, including safety concerns, mistrust of healthcare providers, and misinformation, is crucial for developing effective interventions.

2. Impact of Misinformation: Misinformation and disinformation circulating through traditional and social media platforms contribute to vaccine hesitancy by spreading myths, conspiracy theories, and false claims about vaccine safety and efficacy. Addressing misinformation requires proactive strategies to counter myths, provide accurate information, and build public confidence in vaccination.

3. Psychological and Sociocultural Factors: Vaccine hesitancy is influenced by psychological factors such as risk perception, trust, and cognitive biases, as well as sociocultural factors including religious beliefs, cultural norms, and historical experiences. Tailoring communication and educational interventions to address diverse beliefs and values is essential for promoting vaccine acceptance.

Section 2: Strategies for Addressing Vaccine Hesitancy

1. Communication and Education Campaigns: Evidence-based communication strategies, including health education campaigns, social

marketing, and community engagement initiatives, can effectively address vaccine hesitancy by providing accurate information, dispelling myths, and building trust in vaccination. Culturally sensitive and linguistically appropriate messaging enhances relevance and effectiveness.

2. Healthcare Provider Training: Healthcare providers play a critical role in addressing vaccine hesitancy through effective communication, counseling, and recommendation of vaccines. Training programs that enhance providers' knowledge, communication skills, and confidence in addressing vaccine concerns empower them to engage with hesitant individuals and address their questions and concerns.

3. Multi-Stakeholder Collaboration: Collaborative efforts involving healthcare professionals, public health authorities, community leaders, advocacy groups, and media organizations are essential for addressing vaccine hesitancy comprehensively. Multi-stakeholder partnerships facilitate coordinated communication, resource sharing,

and advocacy for vaccination, amplifying the impact of interventions.

4. Regulation and Policy Interventions: Regulatory measures and policy interventions can help mitigate the spread of vaccine misinformation and promote vaccine acceptance. Measures such as regulating advertising of unproven remedies, combating online misinformation, and enforcing vaccination requirements for certain activities contribute to a supportive environment for vaccination.

5. Community Engagement and Empowerment: Engaging communities in decision-making processes, empowering individuals to make informed choices about vaccination, and addressing underlying social determinants of health are key components of comprehensive strategies to address vaccine hesitancy. Community-led initiatives, peer support networks, and participatory approaches foster trust, resilience, and vaccine confidence at the grassroots level.

....

Chapter 5: The Future of Immunization: Innovations and Challenges

Advances in Vaccine Development

1. Next-Generation Vaccines: Emerging technologies such as mRNA vaccines, viral vector vaccines, and nanoparticle-based vaccines offer promising avenues for developing novel vaccines with improved efficacy, safety, and scalability. These innovative platforms enable rapid vaccine development and customization, facilitating responses to evolving infectious disease threats.

2. Targeted Vaccines for Global Health Priorities: Research efforts are focused on developing vaccines targeting priority global health challenges, including emerging infectious diseases, antimicrobial resistance, and neglected tropical diseases. Targeted vaccine development initiatives aim to address

unmet medical needs and improve health outcomes in vulnerable populations worldwide.

3. Vaccine Delivery Systems: Innovations in vaccine delivery technologies, such as microneedle patches, needle-free injectors, and oral delivery systems, enhance vaccine accessibility, acceptability, and effectiveness. These advancements optimize vaccine administration, reduce reliance on cold chain storage, and facilitate mass vaccination campaigns in resource-limited settings.

4. Adjuvants and Vaccine Formulation: Adjuvants and vaccine formulation strategies play a crucial role in enhancing vaccine immunogenicity, durability, and cross-reactivity. Research into novel adjuvants and formulation approaches aims to optimize vaccine-induced immune responses, improve vaccine stability, and broaden vaccine coverage against diverse pathogens.

5. Personalized Vaccines and Precision Immunization: Advances in immunogenetics, systems biology, and computational modeling enable personalized vaccine development and

precision immunization strategies tailored to individual immune profiles, genetic susceptibilities, and epidemiological contexts. Precision vaccinology approaches optimize vaccine effectiveness, minimize adverse reactions, and enhance population-level immunity.

Challenges in Vaccine Development and Deployment:

1. Scientific Complexity and Uncertainty: Vaccine development is inherently complex and requires rigorous preclinical and clinical testing to ensure safety, efficacy, and regulatory approval. Uncertainty surrounding vaccine development timelines, efficacy against emerging variants, and long-term safety profiles presents challenges for pandemic preparedness and response.

2. Vaccine Hesitancy and Misinformation: Vaccine hesitancy fueled by misinformation, mistrust, and complacency poses significant barriers to achieving high vaccine coverage and population immunity. Addressing vaccine hesitancy requires comprehensive

communication, education, and community engagement efforts to build trust in vaccines and combat misinformation.

3. Access and Equity: Disparities in vaccine access, distribution, and affordability contribute to global health inequities and hinder efforts to achieve universal immunization coverage. Addressing barriers to vaccine access, including supply chain constraints, vaccine nationalism, and socioeconomic disparities, is essential for ensuring equitable vaccine distribution and health outcomes.

4. Regulatory and Logistical Challenges: Regulatory requirements, quality assurance standards, and logistical constraints impact vaccine development, manufacturing, and distribution processes. Streamlining regulatory pathways, enhancing manufacturing capacity, and strengthening supply chain infrastructure are critical for accelerating vaccine deployment and response to public health emergencies.

5. Emerging Infectious Disease Threats: Rapidly evolving infectious disease threats, such as novel viruses, antimicrobial-resistant

pathogens, and zoonotic spillover events, pose ongoing challenges for vaccine development and preparedness. Investing in research and development of broadly protective vaccines, surveillance systems, and pandemic response capabilities is essential for mitigating future infectious disease outbreaks.

… ….. … .

Global Efforts Towards Measles Elimination

1. Measles Elimination Goals: The World Health Organization (WHO) and partners have set ambitious targets for measles elimination, aiming to achieve regional elimination in five of the six WHO regions by 2023 and global measles eradication by 2030. These goals prioritize strengthening routine immunization programs, conducting high-quality supplementary immunization activities, and enhancing measles surveillance and outbreak response efforts.

2. Measles-Rubella Vaccination Strategies:
Many countries have adopted measles-rubella
(MR) vaccination strategies to simultaneously
target both diseases and accelerate progress
towards elimination. MR vaccination
campaigns improve vaccine coverage, reduce
logistical burdens, and enhance
cost-effectiveness, streamlining efforts to
control both measles and rubella transmission.

3. Measles Outbreak Response and Control:
Prompt and coordinated outbreak response is
critical for containing measles transmission and
preventing large-scale outbreaks. Effective
outbreak control measures include rapid case
detection and laboratory confirmation,
vaccination of susceptible populations,
implementation of infection control measures,
and community engagement to enhance vaccine
acceptance and coverage.

4. Strengthening Immunization Systems:
Sustainable measles elimination requires
strengthening immunization systems to ensure
high vaccine coverage, equitable access to
vaccines, and robust surveillance and
monitoring mechanisms. Investments in health

infrastructure, workforce capacity building, vaccine supply chain management, and public health communication are essential for maintaining progress towards measles elimination goals.

5. Measles Surveillance and Monitoring: Surveillance plays a central role in monitoring progress towards measles elimination, detecting outbreaks, and guiding immunization strategies. Enhanced measles surveillance systems utilize real-time data collection, laboratory testing, and epidemiological analysis to inform decision-making, identify high-risk populations, and target interventions for maximum impact.

6. Global Measles and Rubella Strategic Plan: The Measles & Rubella Initiative, a global partnership led by WHO, UNICEF, CDC, and other organizations, coordinates efforts to accelerate measles and rubella control and elimination worldwide. The Global Measles and Rubella Strategic Plan 2021-2030 outlines key strategies, priorities, and targets for achieving regional elimination and global eradication of measles and rubella.

7. Multisectoral Collaboration and Advocacy: Measles elimination requires multisectoral collaboration and advocacy to mobilize political commitment, secure funding, and engage stakeholders across health, education, and community sectors. Advocacy efforts raise awareness of the importance of measles vaccination, promote investment in immunization programs, and mobilize resources to support measles elimination initiatives.

....

Conclusion: Charting the Path Forward Reflections on Measles Eradication Efforts

In conclusion, the journey towards measles eradication is marked by significant progress, ongoing challenges, and a shared commitment to safeguarding global health. As we reflect on the achievements and lessons learned from past efforts, it is clear that concerted action and sustained investment are essential for overcoming remaining barriers and achieving our goal of a measles-free world.

While the road ahead may be daunting, it is also paved with opportunities to innovate, collaborate, and advocate for change. By leveraging scientific advancements, strengthening health systems, and addressing social and cultural determinants of health, we can chart a course towards a future where measles is no longer a threat to our communities.

As we navigate the complexities of measles elimination, it is crucial to remain vigilant, adaptable, and inclusive in our approach. Every individual, organization, and country has a role to play in this collective endeavor, and together, we can turn the tide against measles and ensure a healthier, safer world for future generations.

In the spirit of solidarity and shared responsibility, let us commit ourselves to the task at hand, knowing that our efforts today will shape the trajectory of measles eradication tomorrow. Together, we can chart the path forward towards a world where measles is consigned to the annals of history, and every child has the opportunity to thrive, free from the threat of this preventable disease.

…… … ….

Recommendations for Sustainable Immunization Programs

To ensure the sustainability of immunization programs and further progress towards measles eradication, several recommendations can be considered:

1. Strengthen Health Systems: Invest in robust health systems that can deliver immunization services effectively and efficiently. This includes training healthcare workers, improving cold chain storage and logistics, and ensuring access to vaccines in remote or underserved areas.

2. Community Engagement: Foster community involvement and ownership of immunization

programs through outreach, education, and communication initiatives. Engage community leaders, religious institutions, and local organizations to build trust, address misconceptions, and promote vaccine acceptance.

3. Integration of Services: Integrate measles vaccination with other healthcare services, such as routine immunization, maternal and child health programs, and primary care services. This approach maximizes resources, improves coverage, and enhances the overall health impact of immunization efforts.

4. Surveillance and Monitoring: Strengthen disease surveillance systems to detect measles cases promptly, monitor vaccination coverage, and track progress towards elimination goals. Utilize real-time data and innovative technologies to identify outbreaks early and respond rapidly.

5. Equity and Access: Ensure equitable access to vaccines and immunization services for all populations, regardless of socioeconomic status, geographic location, or other demographic

factors. Address barriers to access, such as cost, transportation, and cultural beliefs, to reach vulnerable and marginalized communities.

6. Sustainable Financing: Secure long-term funding commitments for immunization programs from governments, donors, and international partners. Develop innovative financing mechanisms, such as vaccine bonds or social impact investments, to mobilize resources and sustain funding for vaccination efforts.

7. Research and Development: Invest in research and development to improve existing vaccines, develop new vaccines, and advance scientific knowledge on measles transmission, immunity, and control strategies. Support research on vaccine delivery technologies, immunization schedules, and vaccine safety to optimize program effectiveness.

8. Advocacy and Policy Support: Advocate for strong political commitment, policy implementation, and legislative support for immunization at the national and global levels. Engage policymakers, stakeholders, and the

public to prioritize immunization as a key component of public health and sustainable development agendas.

By prioritizing these recommendations and adopting a comprehensive, multi-sectoral approach to immunization, countries can build resilient and sustainable immunization programs that protect populations from measles and other vaccine-preventable diseases, contribute to improved health outcomes, and advance progress towards global health security and equity.